ALL YOU NEED TO KNOW THE PLANT-BASED DIET

A Simple Cookbook Full of Healthy Recipes That Are the Alpha and the Omega of Plant-Based Cuisine

Botanika Green Way

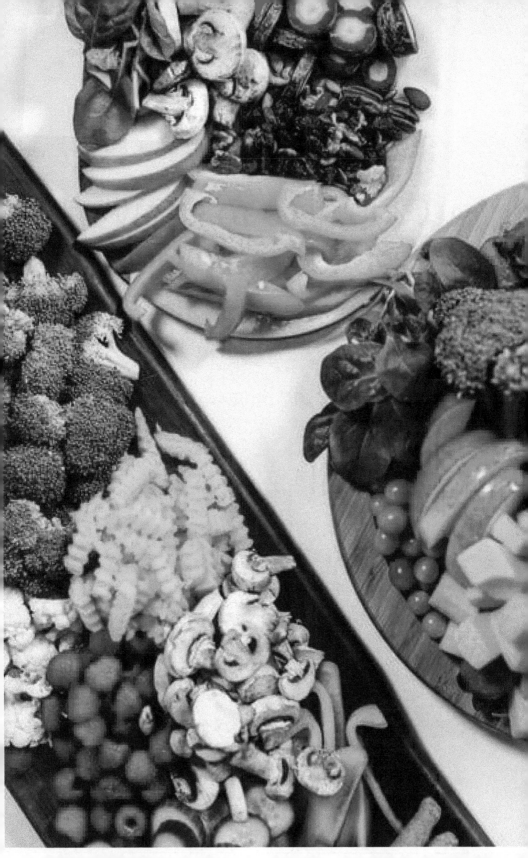

Table of Contents

INTRODUCTION

A plant-based diet is a diet based primarily on whole plant foods. Hence, it excludes animal-sourced foods, hydrogenated oils, refined sugars, and processed foods. A whole food plant-based diet does not consist solely of fruits and vegetables. It includes unprocessed or barely processed oils with healthy fats like extra-virgin olive oil, whole grains, legumes, seeds, and nuts, as well as herbs and spices.

What is the Plant-Based Diet?

The plant-based diet may seem similar to a vegetarian or vegan diet, but it is neither. It's not a diet but a healthy lifestyle. It uses food from plants, and it excludes processed foods like white rice and added sugars, which are allowed in vegan and vegetarian diets.

A plant-based diet is not a diet; it's a healthy way of life

The secret to a healthy diet is simpler than you ever thought! When following a plant-based dietary regimen, you should focus on plant-based foods and avoid animal-sourced food. Whether you are already following a vegan diet or are considering trying this lifestyle, this plant-based, budget-friendly food list makes your grocery shopping easy to manage.

- **VEGETABLES**

Try to include different types of vegetables in your diet from above-ground vegetables to root vegetables, which grow underground.

- **FRUITS**

Choose affordable fruits that are in season. Add frozen fruit to your grocery list since they are just as nutritious as fresh produce. They can be used in smoothies, toppings, compotes, or preserves. On the other hand, dried fruit generally contains a lot of antioxidants, especially polyphenols. It has been proven that eating dried fruits can prevent heart disease and some types of cancer.

- **NUTS & SEEDS**

Nuts and seeds offer different dietary benefits. They do not only ensure essential nutrients but are also offer a variety of flavors. This "ready to eat" food is a perfect snack with dried fruits and trail mix, essential vegan foods to stockpile for an emergency.

- **RICE & GRAINS**

Rice and grains are versatile and easy to incorporate into your diet. Leftovers reheat wonderfully and can be served at any time of the day, turning simple and inexpensive ingredients into a full-fledged meal. You can also make healthy nut butters such as tahini or peanut butter.

- **BEANS & LEGUMES**

Legumes and beans are highly affordable, and there's no end to the variety of tasty dishes you can cook with them. These humble but powerful foods are packed with vitamins, minerals, protein, and dietary fiber. In addition to being super-healthy and versatile, legumes pair very well with other proteins, vegetables, and grains.

- **HEALTHY FATS**

Don't underestimate the importance of quality fats in cooking. Coconut oil, olive oil, and avocado are always good to have on hand.

- **NON-DAIRY PRODUCTS**

Using a plant-based cheese or milk lends flavor, texture, and nutrition to your meals. You can find fantastic products on the market, and this book has many wonderful recipes for feta, vegan ricotta, and plant-based milk.

- **HERBS, SPICES & CONDIMENTS**

A handful of fresh herbs will add that little something extra to your soups, stews, dips, or casseroles. Condiments such as mustard, ketchup, vegan mayonnaise, and plant-based sauces can be used in salads, casseroles, and spreads. Choosing their distinctive flavors to complement vegetables, grains and legumes will help you to make the most of your vegan dishes. Herbs and spices are naturally plant-based, but play it safe and look for a label that says *Vegan-friendly.*

- **BAKING GOODS & CANNED GOODS**

These vegan essentials include all types of flour, baking powder, baking soda, and yeast. Further, cocoa powder, vegan chocolate, and sweeteners are good to have on hand. As for the healthy vegan sweeteners, opt for fresh or dried fruits, agave syrup, maple syrup, and stevia. When it comes to canned goods, stock your pantry with cooking essentials such as tomato, sauerkraut, pickles, low sodium chickpeas and beans, coconut milk, green chilies, pumpkin puree, tomato sauce, low sodium corn, and artichoke hearts. Thus, if you want to make sure you have nutritious, delicious, and quality meals for you and your family, having a vegan pantry is halfway there.

Why You Ought to Reduce Your Intake of Processed and Animal-Based Foods

You have heard over and over that processed food has adverse effects on your health. You might have also been told repeatedly to stay away from foods with lots of preservatives. However, you may have never heard any genuine or concrete facts about why these foods are unsafe. Consequently, let us properly dissect it to help you properly comprehend why you ought to stay away from these offenders.

- **They have massive habit-forming characteristics**

Humans have a predisposition toward being addicted to some specific foods; however, the reality is that the fault is not wholly ours.

Every one of the unhealthy treats we relish now and then triggers a dopamine release. This creates a pleasurable effect in our brain, but the excitement is usually short-lived. The discharged dopamine gradually causes an attachment, and this is the reason some people consistently go back to eat certain unhealthy foods even when they know they're unhealthy and unnecessary. You can get rid of this by avoiding the temptation completely.

- **They are sugar-laden and heavy in glucose-fructose syrup**

Animal-based and processed foods are laden with refined sugars and glucose-fructose syrup, which has almost no nutritional value. An ever-increasing number of studies are affirming what several people presumed from the start: that genetically modified foods bring about inflammatory bowel disease, which consequently makes it increasingly difficult for the body to assimilate essential nutrients. The disadvantages that result from your body being unable to assimilate essential nutrients from consumed foods rightly cannot be overemphasized.

Processed and animal-based food products contain plenteous amounts of refined carbohydrates. Indeed, your body requires carbohydrates to give it energy to function.

In any case, refining carbs dispenses with the fundamental supplements in the way that refining entire grains disposes of the whole grain part. What remains in the wake of refining is what's considered empty carbs or empty calories. These can negatively affect the metabolic system in your body by sharply increasing your blood sugar and insulin levels.

- **They contain lots of synthetic ingredients**

When your body takes in non-natural ingredients, it regards them as a foreign substance and a health threat. It isn't accustomed to identifying synthetic compounds like sucralose or synthesized sugars. Hence, in defense of your health against this foreign "aggressor," your body does what it's programmed to do to safeguard your health: It sets off an immune reaction to tackle this "enemy" compound, which indirectly weakens your body's general disease alertness, making you susceptible to illnesses. The energy expended by your body in triggering your immune system could be better utilized somewhere else.

- **They contain constituent elements that set off a sensation in your body**

A part of processed and animal-based foods contains compounds like glucose-fructose syrup, monosodium glutamate, and specific food dyes that can trigger some addictions. They teach your body to receive a benefit whenever you consume them. Monosodium glutamate, for example, is added to many store-bought baked foods. This additive slowly conditions your palate to relish and crave the taste.

- **This reward-centric arrangement makes you crave it increasingly, which ends up exposing you to the danger of over-consuming calories**

For animal protein, usually, the expression "subpar" is used to allude to plant proteins since they generally have lower levels of essential amino acids as against animal-sourced protein. Nevertheless, what the vast majority don't know is that large amounts of essential amino acids can prove detrimental to your health. Let me break it down further for you.

- **Animal-sourced protein has no fiber**

In their pursuit to consume animal protein, the vast majority wind up dislodging the plant protein that was previously available in their body. Replacing the plant proteins with its animal variant is harmful because, in contrast to plant protein, animal proteins typically are deficient in fiber, phyto-nutrients, and antioxidant properties. Fiber insufficiency is a regular feature across various regions and societies on the planet. In America, for example, according to the National Academy of Medicine, the typical adult takes in roughly 15 grams of dietary fiber daily rather than the recommended daily quantity of 25 to 30 grams. A deficiency in dietary fiber often leads to a heightened risk of breast and colorectal cancers, in addition to constipation, inflammatory bowel disease, and cardiovascular disease.

- **Animal protein brings about an upsurge in phosphorus levels in the body**

Animal protein has significant levels of phosphorus. Our bodies stabilize these plenteous amounts of phosphorus by producing and discharging a hormone known as fibroblast growth factor 23 (FGF23). Studies have shown that this hormone is dangerous to our veins. FGF23 also causes asymmetrical expansion of heart muscles—a determinant for congestive heart failure and even mortality in some advanced cases.

Having discussed the many problems associated with animal protein, it becomes more apt to replace its "high quality" perception with the tag "highly hazardous." In contrast to caffeine, which has a withdrawal effect if it's discontinued abruptly, you can stop taking processed and animal-based foods right away without any withdrawals. Possibly the only thing that you'll give up is the ease of some meals taking little to no time to prepare.

Health Benefits of the Plant-Based Diet

Plant-based eating is one of the healthiest diets in the world. It should include plenty of fresh products, whole grains, legumes, and healthy fats such as seeds and nuts, which are rich in antioxidants, minerals, vitamins, and dietary fiber.

Scientific research has shown that higher use of plant-based foods is connected to a lower risk of death from conditions such as cardiovascular disease, diabetes, hypertension, and obesity. Vegan eating relies heavily on healthy staples, avoiding animal products. Animal products contain much more fat than plant-based foods; it's not a shocker that studies have shown that meat-eaters have nine times the obesity rate of vegans.

This leads us to the next point, one of the greatest benefits of the vegan diet: weight loss. While many people choose to live a vegan life for ethical reasons, the diet itself can help you achieve your weight loss goals. If you're struggling to shift pounds, you may want to consider trying a plant-based diet. How exactly? As a vegan, you will reduce the number of high-calorie foods such as full-fat dairy products, fatty fish, pork, and other cholesterol-containing foods such as eggs. Try replacing such foods with high-fiber and protein-rich alternatives that will keep you fuller longer. The key is focusing on nutrient-dense, clean and natural foods and avoiding empty calories such as sugar, saturated fats, and highly processed foods. Here are a few tricks that help me maintain my weight on the vegan diet. I eat vegetables as a main course; I consume good fats in moderation (good fats such as olive oil do not make you fat); I exercise regularly and cook at home. Plant foods are an excellent source of many nutrients that boost the body's metabolism in many ways. They are easy to digest thanks to their rich content of antioxidants.

- **Reduced Risk of Heart Diseases**

Processed and animal foods are responsible for much heart disease. A whole foods plant-based diet is better at nourishing the body with essential nutrients while improving the heart's function to produce and transport blood to and from the various body parts.

- **Prevents and Heals Diabetes**

Plant-based foods are excellent at reducing high blood sugar. Many studies comparing a vegetarian and vegan diet to a regular meat-filled diet proved that dieting with more plant foods reduced the risk of diabetes by 50 percent.

- **Improved Cognitive Incline**

Fruits and vegetables are excellent for cleansing and boosting metabolism. They release high numbers of plant compounds and antioxidants that slow or prevent cognitive decline. On a plant-based diet, the brain is boosted with sustainable energy, promoting sharp memory, language, thinking, and judgment abilities.

- **Quick Weight Loss**

A high animal food diet is known to drive weight gain. Switching to a plant-based diet helps the body shed fat walls easily, which quickly drives weight loss.

BREAKFAST

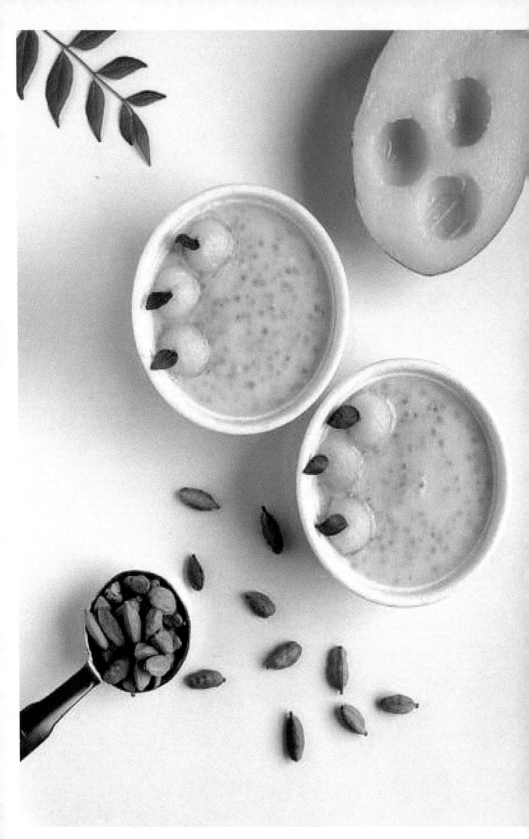

Scrambled Tofu with Bell Pepper

6 Servings

Preparation Time: 20 minutes

Ingredients

- 2 tbsps Plant butter, for frying
- 1 green Bell pepper, chopped
- 1 Tomato, finely chopped
- 2 tbsps chopped fresh Green onions
- Salt and Black pepper to taste
- 1 tsp Turmeric powder
- 1 tsp Creole Seasoning
- ½ cup chopped Baby kale
- 1 (14 oz) pack firm Tofu, crumbled
- 1 red Bell pepper, chopped
- ¼ cup grated plant-based Parmesan

Directions

- Melt the plant butter in a pan over medium heat and add the tofu.

- Cook with occasional stirring until the tofu is light golden brown while, make sure not to break the tofu into tiny bits but to have scrambled egg resemblance, for 5 minutes.

- Stir in the bell peppers, tomato, green onions, salt, black pepper, turmeric powder, and Creole seasoning.

- Sauté until the vegetables soften for 5 minutes.

- Mix in the kale to wilt, 3 minutes, and then half of the plant-based Parmesan cheese.

- Allow melting for 1 to 2 minutes, and then turn the heat off. Top with the remaining cheese and serve warm.

Veggie Panini

6 Servings

Preparation Time: 30 minutes

Ingredients

- 1 tbsp Olive oil
- 1 ripe avocado, sliced
- 2 tbsps freshly squeezed Lemon juice
- 1 tbsp chopped parsley
- ½ tsp pure Maple syrup
- 8 slices Whole-wheat ciabatta
- 1 cup sliced button Mushrooms
- Salt and Black pepper to taste
- 4 oz sliced plant-based Parmesan

Directions and

- Heat the olive oil in a medium pan over medium heat and sauté the mushrooms until softened, for 5 minutes.

- Season with salt and black pepper. Turn the heat off.

- Preheat a panini press to medium heat, 3 to 5 minutes.

- Mash the avocado in a medium bowl and mix in lemon juice, parsley, and maple syrup.

- Spread the mixture on 4 bread slices, divide the mushrooms and plant-based Parmesan cheese on top.

- Cover with the other bread slices and brush the top with olive oil.

- Grill the sandwiches one after another in the heated press until golden brown and the cheese is melted. Serve.

Cheddar Grits with Soy Chorizo

8 Servings

Preparation Time: 25 minutes

Ingredients

- 1 cup quick-cooking Grits
- 2 tbsps Peanut butter
- 1 cup Soy chorizo, chopped
- 1 cup Corn kernels
- ½ cup grated plant-based Cheddar
- 2 cups vegetable broth

Directions

- Preheat oven to 380°F.

- Add the broth into a pot and bring to a boil over medium heat.

- Stir in salt and grits. Lower the heat and cook until the grits are thickened, stirring often.

- Turn the heat off, put in the plant-based cheddar cheese, peanut butter, soy chorizo, and corn and mix well.

- Spread the mixture into a greased baking dish and bake for 45 minutes until slightly puffed and golden brown. Serve right away.

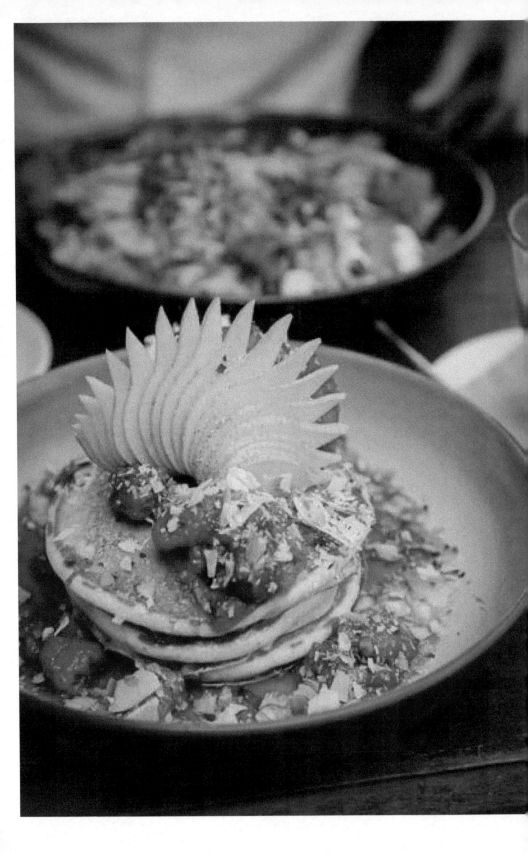

Vanilla Crepes with Berry Cream Compote Topping

6 Servings

Preparation Time: 35 minutes

Ingredients

For the berry cream

- 2 tbsps Plant butter
- 1 tsp Vanilla extract
- ½ cup fresh Blueberries
- ½ cup fresh Raspberries
- 2 tbsps pure Date sugar
- ½ cup whipped Coconut cream

For the crepes

- 2 tbsps Flax seed powder
- 1 tsp pure Date sugar
- ¼ tsp Salt
- 2 cups Almond flour
- 1 ½ cups Almond milk
- 1 ½ cups Water
- 1 tsp Vanilla extract
- 3 tbsps Plant butter for frying

Directions

- Melt butter in a pot over low heat and mix in the date sugar and vanilla.

- Cook until the sugar melts, and then toss in berries. Allow softening for 2-3 minutes. Set aside to cool.

- In a medium bowl, mix the flax seed powder with 6 tbsps water and allow it to thicken for about 5 minutes to make the vegan "flax egg."

- Whisk in vanilla, date sugar, and salt. Pour in a quarter cup of almond flour and whisk, then a quarter cup of almond milk, and mix until no lumps remain.

- Repeat the mixing process with the remaining almond flour and almond milk in the same quantities.

- Mix in 1 cup of water until the mixture is runny like that of pancakes, and add the remaining water until it is lighter.

- Brush a large non-stick pan with some butter and place over medium heat to melt.

- Add 1 tablespoon of the batter into the pan and swirl the pan quickly and all around to coat the pan with the batter.

- Cook until the batter is dry and golden brown beneath, about 30 seconds.

- Use a spatula to carefully flip the crepe and cook the other side until golden brown too. Fold the crepe onto a plate and set it aside.

- Repeat making more crepes with the remaining batter until exhausted.

- Plate the crepes, top with the whipped coconut cream and the berry compote. Serve immediately.

Morning Naan Bread with Mango Jam

6 Servings

Preparation Time: 40 minutes

Ingredients

- ¾ cup Almond flour
- 1/3 cup Olive oil
- 2 cups boiling water
- 2 tbsps Plant butter for frying
- 4 cups heaped chopped Mangoes
- 1 cup pure Maple syrup
- 1 Lemon, juiced
- A pinch of Saffron powder
- 1 tsp Salt + extra for sprinkling
- 1 tsp Baking powder
- 1 tsp Cardamom powder

Directions

- In a large bowl, mix the almond flour, salt, and baking powder.

- Mix in the olive oil and boiling water until smooth, thick batter forms. Allow the dough to rise for about 5 minutes.

- Make balls out of the dough, put each on baking paper, and use your hands to flatten the dough.

- Melt the plant butter in a large pan and fry the dough on both sides until set and golden brown on each side, for 4 minutes per bread.

- Transfer to a plate and set aside for serving.

- Add the mangoes, maple syrup, lemon juice, and 3 tbsps water in a pot and cook until boiling for 5 minutes.

- Mix in saffron and cardamom powders and cook further over low heat until the mangoes soften.

- Mash the mangoes with the back of the spoon until relatively smooth with little chunks of mangoes in a jam.

- Cool completely. Spoon the jam into sterilized jars and serve with the naan bread.

Crispy Corn Cakes

6 Servings

Preparation Time: 35 minutes

Ingredients

- 1 tbsp Flaxseed powder
- 1 tsp Salt
- 2 tsps Baking powder
- 4 tbsps Olive oil
- 2 cups yellow Cornmeal
- 1 cup Tofu mayonnaise for serving

Directions

- In a bowl, mix the flax seed powder with 3 tbsps water and allow thickening for 5 minutes to form the vegan "flax egg."

- Add in 1 cup of water and then whisk in the cornmeal, salt, and baking powder until soup texture forms but not watery.

- Warm a quarter of the olive oil in a griddle pan and pour in a quarter of the batter. Cook until set and golden brown beneath, for 3 minutes.

- Flip the cake and cook the other side until set and golden brown too.

- Plate the cake and make three more with the remaining oil and batter.

- Top the cakes with some tofu mayonnaise before serving.

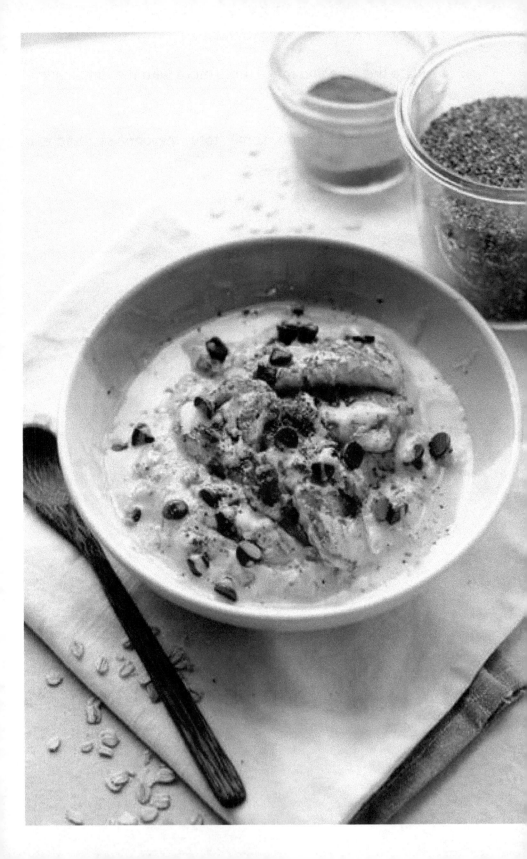

Coconut Chia Pudding

6 Servings

Preparation Time: 5 minutes+ cooling time

Ingredients

- 1 cup Coconut milk
- 3 tbsps Chia seeds
- ½ cup Granola
- ½ tsp Vanilla extract
- 2/3 cup chopped sweet Nectarine

Directions

- In a medium bowl, mix the coconut milk, vanilla, and chia seeds until well combined.

- Divide the mixture between 6 breakfast cups and refrigerate for at least 4 hours to allow the mixture to gel.

- Top with the granola and nectarine. Serve.

DRINKS

Chocolate and Cherry Smoothie

2 Servings

Preparation Time: 5 minutes

Ingredients

- 4 cups frozen cherries
- 2 tablespoons cocoa powder
- 1 scoop of protein powder
- 1 teaspoon maple syrup
- 2 cups almond milk, unsweetened

Directions

- Place all the ingredients in the order in a food processor or blender and then pulse for 2 to 3 minutes at high speed until smooth.
- Pour the smoothie into two glasses and then serve.

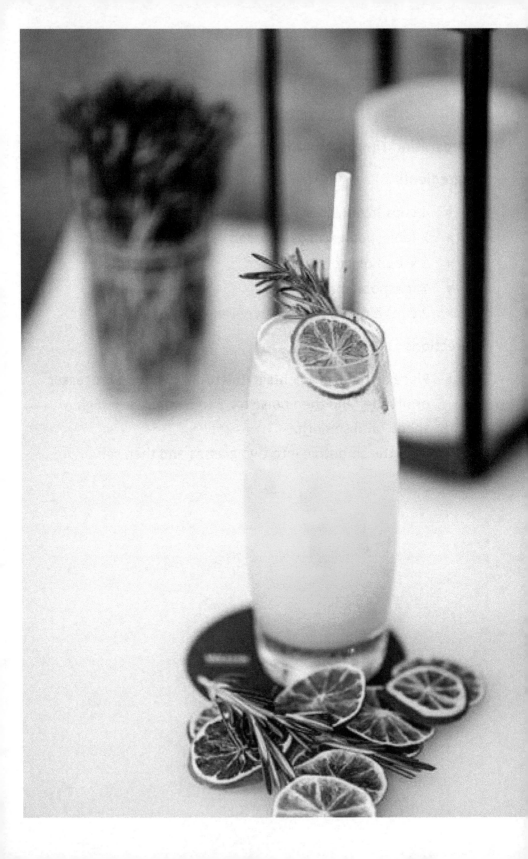

Banana Weight Loss Juice

2 Servings

Preparation Time: 10 minutes

Ingredients

- 1/3 Cup Water
- 1 Apple, Sliced
- 1 Orange, Sliced
- 1 Banana, Sliced
- 1 tablespoon Lemon Juice

Directions

- Simply place everything into your blender, blend on high for twenty seconds, and then pour into your glass.

Vitamin Green Smoothie

2 Servings

Preparation Time: 5 minutes

Ingredients

- 1 cup milk or juice
- 1 cup spinach or kale
- ½ cup plain yogurt
- 1 kiwi
- 1 Tbsp chia or flax
- 1 tsp vanilla

Directions

- Mix the milk or juice and greens until smooth. Add the remaining ingredients and continue blending until smooth again.
- Enjoy your delicious drink!

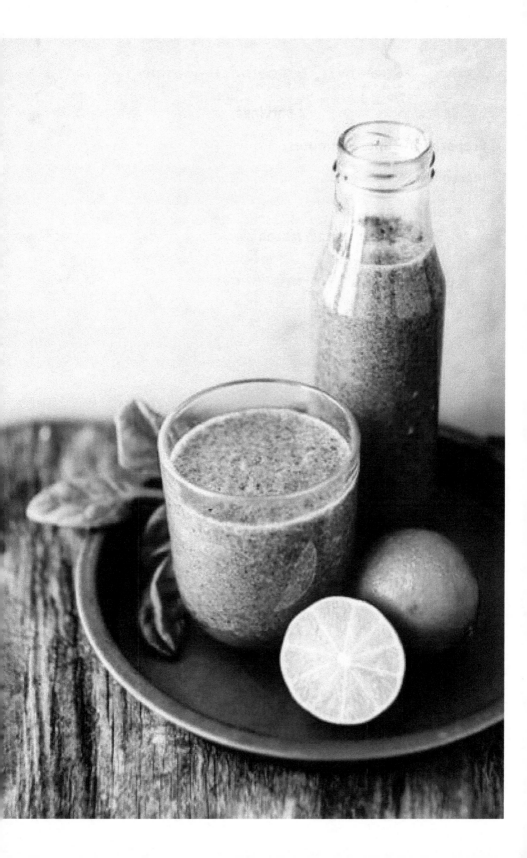

Strawberry Grapefruit Smoothie

2 Servings

Preparation Time: 5 minutes

Ingredients

- 1 banana
- ½ cup strawberries, frozen
- 1 grapefruit
- ¼ cup milk
- ¼ cup plain yogurt
- 2 tbsps honey
- ½ tsp ginger, chopped

Directions

- Using a mixer, blend all the ingredients.
- When smooth, top your drink with a slice of grapefruit and enjoy it!

Brownie Batter Orange Chia Shake

2 Servings

Preparation Time: 5 minutes

Ingredients

- 2 tablespoons cocoa powder
- 3 tablespoons chia seeds
- ¼ teaspoon salt
- 4 tablespoons chocolate chips
- 4 teaspoons coconut sugar
- ½ teaspoon orange zest
- ½ teaspoon vanilla extract, unsweetened
- 2 cups almond milk

Directions

- Place all the ingredients in the order in a food processor or blender and then pulse for 2 to 3 minutes at high speed until smooth.
- Pour the smoothie into two glasses and then serve.

LUNCH

Roasted Butternut Squash with Chimichurri

6 Servings

Preparation Time: 15 minutes

Ingredients

- Zest and juice of 1Llemon
- ½ cup chopped fresh Parsley
- 2 Garlic cloves, minced
- 1 lb butternut squash
- 1 tbsp plant butter, melted
- 3 tbsps toasted Pine nuts
- ½ medium red Bell pepper, chopped
- 1 Jalapeno pepper, chopped
- 1 cup Olive oil

Directions

- Add the lemon zest and juice, red bell pepper, jalapeno, olive oil, parsley, garlic, salt, and black pepper in a bowl.

- Use an immersion blender to grind the ingredients until your desired consistency is achieved; set aside the chimichurri.

- Slice the butternut squash into rounds and remove the seeds.

- Drizzle with the plant butter and season with salt and black pepper.

- Preheat a grill pan over medium heat and cook the squash for 2 minutes on each side or until browned.

- Remove the squash to serving plates, scatter the pine nuts on top, and serve with the chimichurri and red cabbage salad.

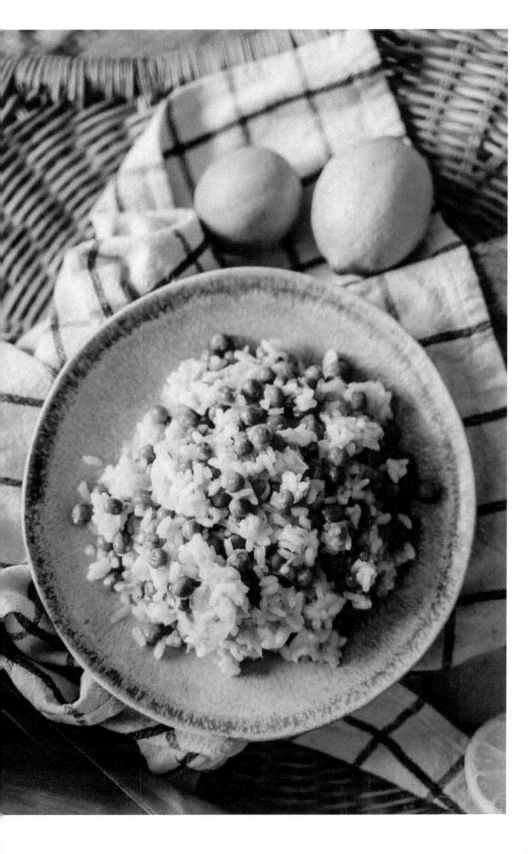

Sweet and Spicy Brussel Sprout Stir-Fry

6 Servings

Preparation Time: 15 minutes

Ingredients

- 4 oz plant Butter + more to taste
- Hot Chili sauce
- 4 shallots, chopped
- 1 tbsp apple cider Vinegar
- Salt and Black pepper to taste
- 1 lb Brussels sprouts

Directions

- Add the plant butter in a saucepan and melt over medium heat.

- Pour in the shallots and sauté for 2 minutes, to caramelize and slightly soften. Add the apple cider vinegar, salt, and black pepper.

- Stir and reduce the heat to cook the shallots further with continuous stirring, about 5 minutes. Transfer to a plate after.

- Trim the Brussel sprouts and cut them in halves.

- Leave the small ones as wholes. Pour the Brussel sprouts into the saucepan and stir-fry with more plant butter until softened but al dente.

- Season with salt and black pepper, stir in the onions and hot chili sauce, and heat for a few seconds. Serve immediately.

Black Bean Burgers with BBQ Sauce

6 Servings

Preparation Time: 20 minutes

Ingredients

- 3 (15 oz) cans black beans, drained
- 2 tbsps whole-wheat flour
- 2 tbsps quick-cooking oats
- ¼ cup chopped fresh basil
- 2 tbsps pure barbecue sauce
- 1 garlic clove, minced
- Salt and black pepper to taste
- 4 whole-grain hamburger buns, split

For topping
- Red onion slices
- Tomato slices
- Fresh basil leaves
- Additional barbecue sauce

Directions

- In a medium bowl, mash the black beans and mix in the flour, oats, basil, barbecue sauce, garlic salt, and black pepper until well combined. Mold 4 patties out of the mixture and set aside.

- Heat a grill pan to medium heat and lightly grease with cooking spray. Cook the bean patties on both sides until light brown and cooked through, 10 minutes.

- Place the patties between the burger buns and top with the onions, tomatoes, basil, and some barbecue sauce. Serve warm.

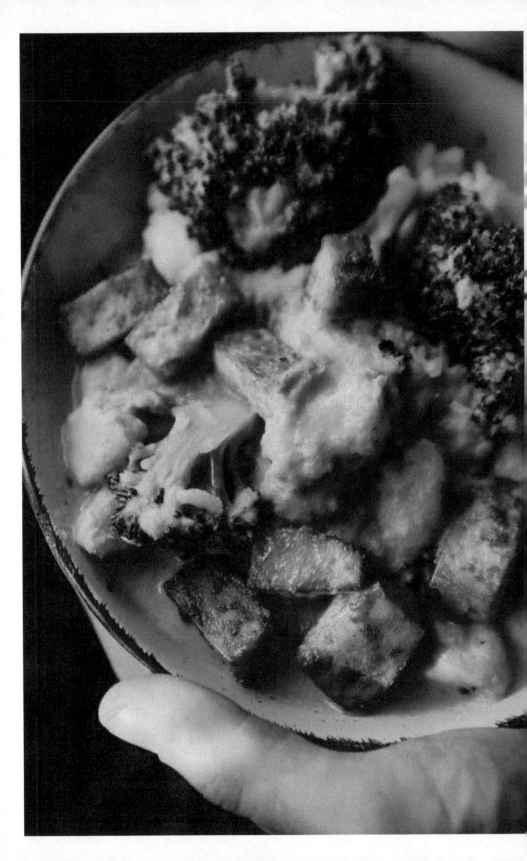

Creamy Brussels sprouts Bake

6 Servings

Preparation Time: 26 minutes

Ingredients

- 3 tbsps plant butter
- 1 ¼ cups coconut cream
- 10 oz grated plant-based mozzarella
- ¼ cup grated plant-based Parmesan
- Salt and black pepper to taste
- 1 cup tempeh, cut into 1-inch cubes
- 1 ½ lbs halved Brussels sprouts
- 5 garlic cloves, minced

Directions

- Preheat oven to 400 F.

- Melt the plant butter in a large skillet over medium heat and fry the tempeh cubes until browned on both sides, about 6 minutes.

- Remove onto a plate and set aside. Pour the Brussels sprouts and garlic into the skillet and sauté until fragrant.

- Mix in coconut cream and simmer for 4 minutes.

- Add tempeh cubes and combine well. Pour the sauté into a baking dish, sprinkle with plant-based mozzarella cheese, and plant-based Parmesan cheese.

- Bake for 10 minutes or until golden brown on top. Serve with tomato salad.

Basil Pesto Seitan Panini

6 Servings

Preparation Time : 15 minutes+ cooling time

Ingredients

For the seitan
- 2/3 cup basil pesto
- 1/8 tsp salt
- 1 cup chopped seitan
- ½ lemon, juiced
- 1 garlic clove, minced

For the panini
- 3 tbsps basil pesto
- 1 yellow bell pepper, chopped
- ¼ cup grated plant Parmesan cheese
- 8 thick slices whole-wheat ciabatta
- Olive oil for brushing
- 8 slices plant-based mozzarella

Directions

- In a medium bowl, mix the pesto, lemon juice, garlic, and salt. Add the seitan and coat well with the marinade. Cover with plastic wrap and marinate in the refrigerator for 30 minutes.

- Preheat a large skillet over medium heat and remove the seitan from the fridge. Cook the seitan in the pan until brown and cooked through, 2-3 minutes. Turn the heat off.

- Preheat a Panini press to medium heat. In a small bowl, mix the pesto in the inner parts of two slices of bread.

- On the outer parts, apply some olive oil and place a slice with (the olive oil side down) in the press. Lay 2 slices of plant-based mozzarella cheese on the bread, spoon some seitan on top.

- Sprinkle with some bell pepper and some plant-based Parmesan cheese. Cover with another bread slice.

- Close the press and grill the bread for 1 to 2 minutes.

- Flip the bread, and grill further for 1 minute or until the cheese melts and golden brown on both sides. Serve warm.

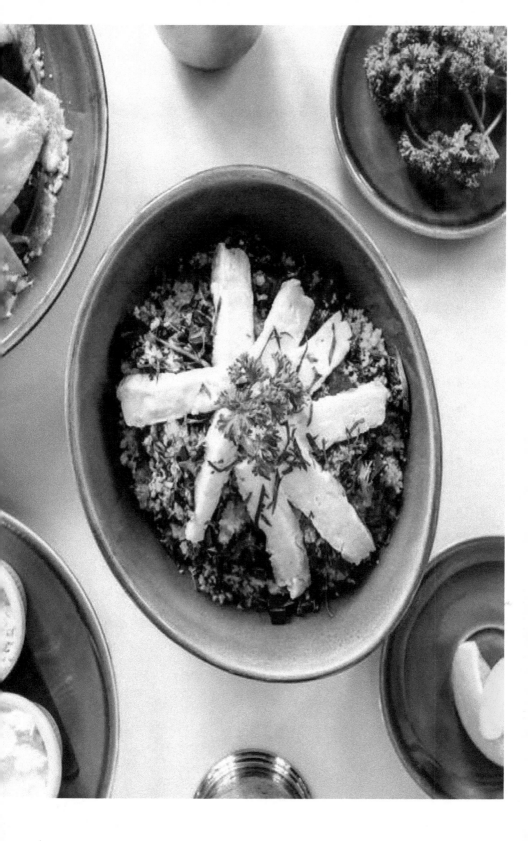

Jalapeño Quinoa Bowl with Lima Beans

6 Servings

Preparation Time: 30 minutes

Ingredients

- 1 tbsp olive oil
- 1 (8 oz) can sweet corn kernels
- 1 (8 oz) can lima beans, rinsed
- 1 cup quick-cooking quinoa
- 1 (14 oz) can diced tomatoes
- 2 ½ cups vegetable broth
- 1 cup grated plant-based cheddar
- 2 tbsps chopped fresh cilantro
- 2 limes, cut into wedges
- 1 avocado, pitted, sliced, and peeled
- 1 lb extra firm tofu, cubed
- Salt and black pepper to taste
- 1 medium yellow onion, finely diced
- ½ cup cauliflower florets
- 1 jalapeño pepper, minced
- 2 garlic cloves, minced
- 1 tbsp red chili powder
- 1 tsp cumin powder

Directions

- Heat olive oil in a pot and cook the tofu until golden brown, 5 minutes. Season with salt, pepper, and mix in onion, cauliflower, and jalapeño pepper.

- Cook until the vegetables soften, 3 minutes.

- Stir in garlic, chili powder, and cumin powder; cook for 1 minute.

- Mix in sweet corn kernels, lima beans, quinoa, tomatoes, and vegetable broth. Simmer until the quinoa absorbs all the liquid, 10 minutes.

- Fluff quinoa. Top with the plant-based cheddar cheese, cilantro, lime wedges, and avocado. Serve.

American-Style Tempeh Bake with Garden Peas

6 Servings

Preparation Time: 50 minutes

Ingredients

- 16 oz whole-wheat bow-tie pasta
- ¼ cup white wine
- ¾ cup vegetable stock
- ¼ cup oats milk
- 2 tsps chopped fresh thyme
- ¼ cup chopped cauliflower
- ½ cup grated plant-based Parmesan
- 3 tbsps whole-wheat breadcrumbs
- 2 tbsps olive oil, divided
- 2/3 lb tempeh, cut into 1-inch cubes
- Salt and black pepper to taste
- 1 medium yellow onion, chopped
- ½ cup sliced white mushrooms
- 2 tbsps whole-wheat flour

Directions

- Cook the pasta in 8 cups of slightly salted water for 10 minutes or until al dente. Drain and set aside.

- Preheat the oven to 375 F. Heat the 1 tbsp of olive oil in a skillet, season the tempeh with salt and pepper, and cook until golden brown all around.

- Mix in onion, mushrooms, and cook for 5 minutes. Stir in flour and cook for 1 more minute.

- Mix in wine and add two-thirds of the vegetable stock.

- Cook for 2 minutes while occasionally stirring and then add milk; continue cooking until the sauce thickens, 4 minutes.

- Season with thyme, salt, black pepper, and half of the Parmesan cheese.

- Once the cheese melts, turn the heat off and allow cooling.

- Add the rest of the vegetable stock and cauliflower to a blender and blend until smooth.

- Pour the mixture into a bowl, add in the sauce, and mix in pasta until combined. Grease a baking dish with cooking spray and spread it in the mixture.

- Drizzle the remaining olive oil on top, breadcrumbs, some more thyme, and remaining cheese.

- Bake until the cheese melts and is golden brown on top, 30 minutes. Remove the dish from the oven, allow cooling for 3 minutes, and serve.

Seitan Cauliflower Gratin

6 Servings

Preparation Time: 40 minutes

Ingredients

- 2 oz plant butter
- 2 cups crumbled seitan
- 1 cup coconut cream
- 2 tbsps mustard powder
- 5 oz grated plant-based Parmesan
- 4 tbsps fresh rosemary
- Salt and black pepper to taste
- 1 leek, coarsely chopped
- 1 white onion, coarsely chopped
- 2 cups broccoli florets
- 1 cup cauliflower florets

Directions

- Preheat oven to 450 F.

- Melt half of the plant butter in a pot over medium heat. Add in leek, white onion, broccoli, and cauliflower and cook for about 6 minutes.

- Transfer the vegetables to a baking dish.

- Melt the remaining butter in a pan over medium heat and cook the seitan until browned.

- Mix the coconut cream and mustard powder in a bowl.

- Pour the mixture over the vegetables. Scatter the seitan and plant-based Parmesan cheese on top and sprinkle with rosemary, salt, and pepper.

- Bake for 15 minutes. Remove to cool for a few minutes and serve.

SNACKS & SIDES

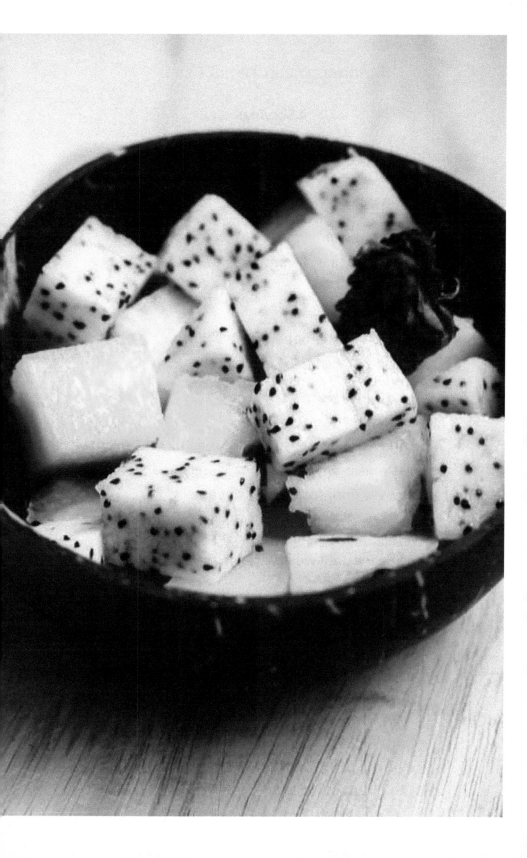

Mediterranean Tahini Beans

4 Servings

Preparation time: 10 minutes

Ingredients

- 1 tbsp sesame oil
- 1 cup string beans, trimmed
- Salt to taste
- 2 tbsps pure tahini
- 2 tbsps coarsely chopped mint leaves
- ¼ tsp red chili flakes for topping

Directions

- Pour the string beans into a medium safe microwave dish, sprinkle with 1 tbsp of water, and steam in the microwave until softened, 1 minute.

- Heat the sesame oil in a large skillet and toss in the string beans until well coated in the butter.

- Season with salt and mix in the tahini and mint leaves.

- Cook for 1 to 2 minutes and turn the heat off. Serve.

Beet & Carrot Stir-Fry

4 Servings

Preparation time: 20 minutes

Ingredients

- 2 beets, peeled and cut into wedges
- 3 small carrots, cut crosswise
- 2 tbsps plant butter
- 1 red onion, cut into wedges
- ½ tsp dried oregano
- 1/8 tsp salt

Directions

- Steam the beets and carrots in a medium safe microwave bowl until softened, 6 minutes.

- Meanwhile, melt the butter in a large skillet and sauté the onion until softened, 3 minutes.

- Stir in the carrots, beets, oregano, and salt. Mix well and cook for 5 minutes. Serve warm.

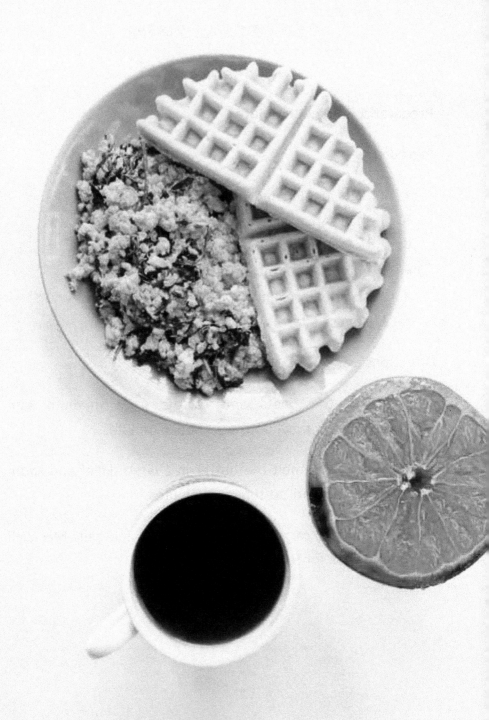

Mustard Tofu-Avocado Wraps

4 Servings

Preparation time: 25 minutes

Ingredients

- 6 tbsps olive oil
- 1 lb extra-firm tofu, cut into strips
- 1 tbsp soy sauce
- ¼ cup apple cider vinegar
- 1 tsp yellow mustard
- 3 cups shredded romaine lettuce
- 3 ripe Roma tomatoes, chopped
- 1 large carrot, shredded
- 1 medium avocado, chopped
- ⅓ cup minced red onion
- ¼ cup sliced pitted green olives
- 4 whole-grain flour tortillas

Directions

- Heat 2 tbsps of olive oil in a skillet over medium heat. Place the tofu, cook for 10 minutes until golden brown.

- Drizzle with soy sauce. Let cool.

- In a bowl, whisk the vinegar, mustard, salt, pepper, and the remaining oil.

- In another bowl, mix the lettuce, tomatoes, carrot, avocado, onion, and olives.

- Pour the dressing over the salad and toss to coat.

- Lay out a tortilla on a clean flat surface and spoon ¼ of the salad, some tofu, and then roll-up. Cut in half.

- Repeat the process with the remaining tortillas. Serve.

Maple-Glazed Butternut Squash

4 Servings

Preparation time: 40 minutes

Ingredients

- 1 butternut squash, cubed
- 2 tbsps olive oil
- 4 garlic cloves, minced
- ¼ cup pure maple syrup
- 1 tsp red chili flakes
- 1 tsp coriander seeds

Directions

- Preheat the oven to 375 F.

- In a medium bowl, toss the squash with olive oil, garlic, maple syrup, salt, black pepper, red chili flakes, and coriander seeds.

- Spread the mixture on a baking sheet and roast in the oven for 25 to 30 minutes or until the potatoes soften and golden brown.

- Remove from the oven, plate, and serve.

Tofu & Tomato Sandwiches

4 Servings

Preparation time: 15 minutes

Ingredients

- 1 lb extra-firm tofu, crumbled
- 1 medium carrot, chopped
- 1 celery stalk, chopped
- 3 green onions, minced
- ¼ cup shelled sunflower seeds
- ½ cup tofu mayonnaise
- 8 slices whole-grain bread
- 4 slices ripe tomato
- 4 lettuce leaves

Directions

- Place the tofu in a bowl.

- Stir in carrot, celery, green onions, and sunflower seeds. Mix in mayonnaise, salt, and pepper.

- Toast the bread slices. Spread the tofu mixture onto 4 bread slices.

- Layer a tomato slice and lettuce leaf. Top each sandwich with a bread slice and cut diagonally. Serve immediately.

Parmesan Baby Potatoes

4 Servings

Preparation time: 20 minutes

Ingredients

- 4 tbsps plant butter, melted
- 4 garlic cloves, minced
- 3 tbsps chopped chives
- Salt and black pepper to taste
- 2 tbsps grated plant-based Parmesan
- 1 ½ lbs baby potatoes

Directions

- Preheat the oven to 400 F.

- In a bowl, mix butter, garlic, chives, salt, pepper, and plant Parmesan cheese.

- Toss the potatoes in the butter mixture until coated. Spread the mixture into a baking sheet, cover with foil, and roast for 30 minutes.

- Remove the potatoes from the oven and toss in the remaining butter mixture. Serve.

Guacamole with Daikon

4 Servings

Preparation time: 15 minutes

Ingredients

- Juice of 1 lime
- 1 avocado, cubed
- ½ red onion, sliced
- 1 garlic clove, minced
- ¼ cup chopped cilantro
- 1 daikon, cut into matchsticks

Directions

- Place the avocado in a bowl and squeeze the lime juice.

- Sprinkle with salt.

- Mash the avocado using a fork, stir in onion, garlic, and cilantro.

- Serve with daikon slices.

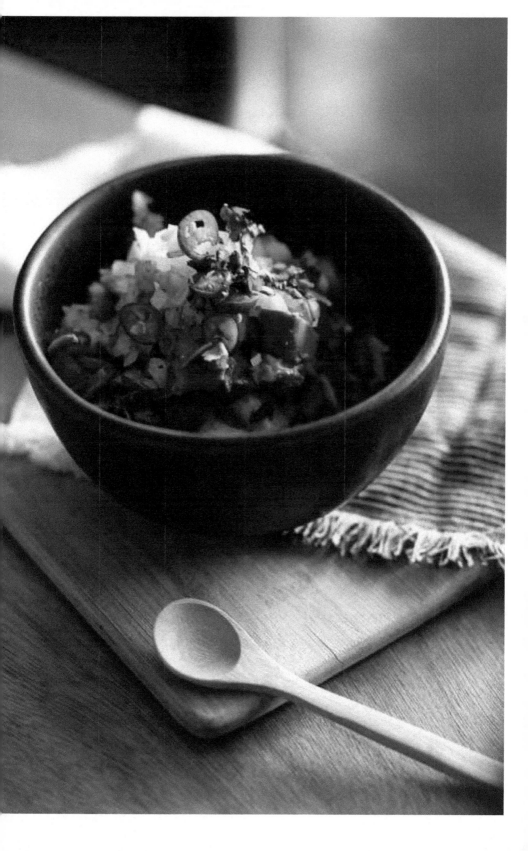

Tofu Stuffed Peppers

8 Servings

Preparation time: 25 minutes

Ingredients

- 2 cups red and yellow bell peppers
- 2 oz tofu, chopped into small bits
- 2 cups cashew cream cheese
- 2 tbsps chili paste, mild
- 4 tbsps melted plant butter
- 2 cups grated plant-based Parmesan

Directions

- Preheat oven to 400 F.

- Use a knife to cut the bell peppers into two (lengthwise) and remove the core.

- In a bowl, mix tofu, cashew cream cheese, chili paste, and melted butter until smooth.

- Spoon the cheese mixture into the bell peppers and use the back of the spoon to level the filling in the peppers.

- Grease a baking sheet with cooking spray and arrange the stuffed peppers on the sheet.

- Sprinkle the plant-based Parmesan cheese on top and bake the peppers for 15-20 minutes until the peppers are golden brown and the cheese melted.

- Remove onto a serving platter and serve warm.

SOUPS & SALADS

Cayenne Pumpkin Soup

8 Servings

Preparation Time: 55 minutes

Ingredients

- 1 (2-pound) Pumpkin, sliced
- 1 head Garlic
- 6 cups water
- Zest and juice of 1 Lime
- ¼ tsp Cayenne pepper
- ½ tsp ground Coriander
- ½ tsp ground Cumin
- Toasted Pumpkin seeds
- 3 tbsps Olive oil
- 1 tsp Salt
- 2 red Bell peppers
- 1 Onion, halved

Directions

- Preheat oven to 350⁰F.

- Brush the pumpkin slices with oil and sprinkle with salt.

- Arrange the slices skin-side-down and on a greased baking dish and bake for 20 minutes.

- Brush the onion with oil. Cut the top of the garlic head and brush with oil.

- When the pumpkin is ready, add in bell peppers, onion, and garlic, and bake for another 10 minutes. Allow cooling.

- Take out the flesh from the pumpkin skin and transfer it to a food processor.

- Cut the pepper roughly, peel and cut the onion, and remove the cloves from the garlic head.

- Transfer to the food processor and pour in the water, lime zest, and lime juice.

- Blend the soup until smooth. If it's very thick, add a bit of water to reach your desired consistency.

- Sprinkle with salt, cayenne, coriander, and cumin. Serve.

Cream Soup of Zucchini with Walnuts

6 Servings

Preparation Time: 45 minutes

Ingredients

- 3 Zucchinis, chopped
- 4 cups Vegetable stock
- 3 tsps ground Sage
- 3 tbsps nutritional yeast
- 1 cup non-dairy milk
- ¼ cup toasted Walnuts
- 2 tsps Olive oil
- Sea salt and Black pepper to taste
- 1 Onion, diced

Directions

- Warm the oil in a pan and place zucchini, onion, salt, and pepper; cook for 5 minutes.

- Pour in vegetable stock and bring to a boil. Lower the heat and simmer for 15 minutes.

- Stir in sage, nutritional yeast, and milk. Purée the soup with a blender until smooth.

- Serve garnished with toasted walnuts and pepper.

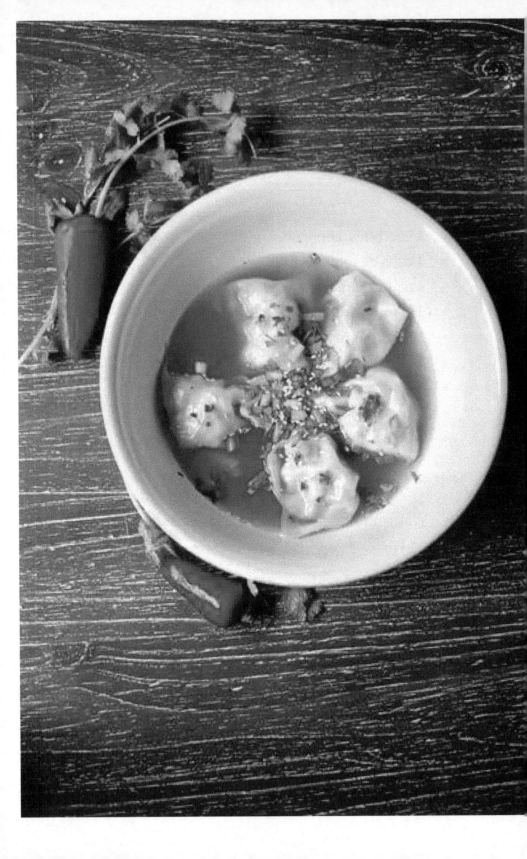

Homemade Ramen Soup

6 Servings

Preparation Time: 25 minutes

Ingredients

- 7 oz Japanese buckwheat noodles
- 1 cup canned Pinto beans, drained
- 2 tbsps fresh Cilantro, chopped
- 2 Scallions, thinly sliced
- 4 tbsps Sesame paste

Directions

- In boiling salted water, add in the noodles and cook for 5 minutes over low heat.

- Remove a cup of the noodle water to a bowl and add in the sesame paste; stir until it has dissolved.

- Pour the sesame mix in the pot with the noodles, add in pinto beans, and stir until everything is hot.

- Serve topped with cilantro and scallions in individual bowls.

Lime Lentil Soup

4 Servings

Preparation Time: 35 minutes

Ingredients

- 1 tsp Olive oil
- 1 cup yellow Lentils
- 1 cup canned crushed Tomatoes
- 2 cups Water
- 1 Celery stalk, chopped
- 2 cups chopped Collard greens
- 1 Onion, chopped
- 6 Garlic cloves, minced
- 1 tsp Chili powder
- ½ tsp ground Cinnamon
- Salt to taste

Directions

- Warm the oil in a pot over medium heat.

- Add the onion and garlic and cook for 5 minutes. Stir in chili powder, celery, cinnamon, and salt. Pour in lentils, tomatoes and juices, and water.

- Bring to a boil, then lower the heat and simmer for 15 minutes.

- Stir in collard greens. Cook for an additional 5 minutes. Serve.

Traditional Lebanese Salad

6 Servings

Preparation Time: 25 minutes

Ingredients

- 1 cup cooked Bulgur
- 1 tbsp Olive oil
- ½ cucumber, sliced
- 1 Tomato, sliced
- 1 cup fresh parsley, chopped
- ¼ cup fresh Mint, chopped
- 2 Scallions, chopped
- 4 tbsps Sunflower seeds
- 1 cup boiling water
- Zest and juice of 1 Lemon
- 1 Garlic clove, pressed
- Sea salt to taste

Directions

- In a bowl, mix the lemon juice, lemon zest, garlic, salt, and olive oil. Stir in cucumber, tomato, parsley, mint, and scallions. Toss to coat.

- Fluff the bulgur and put it into the cucumber mix. Stir to combine.

- Top with sunflower seeds and serve.

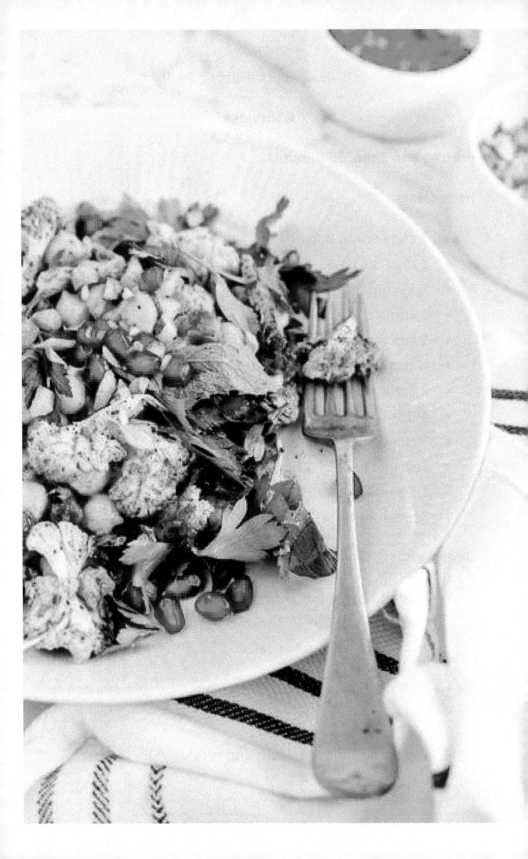

Cucumber, Lettuce & Tomato Salad

6 Servings

Preparation Time: 15 minutes

Ingredients

- ¾ cup Olive oil
- 1 (15.5-oz) can Lentils, drained
- 2 ripe Tomatoes, chopped
- 1 Cucumber, peeled and chopped
- 1 Carrot, chopped
- ½ cup Halved pitted kalamata olives
- 3 small Red radishes, chopped
- 2 tbsps chopped Fresh parsley
- 1 Ripe avocado, chopped
- ¼ cup White wine vinegar
- 2 tsps Dijon mustard
- 1 Garlic clove
- 1 tbsp minced Green onions
- ½ head Romaine lettuce, chopped
- ½ head Iceberg lettuce, chopped

Directions

- Add the oil, vinegar, mustard, garlic, green onions, salt, and pepper in a food processor.

- Pulse until blended. Set aside.

- In a bowl, place the lettuces, lentils, tomatoes, cucumber, carrot, olives, radishes, parsley, and avocado.

- Pour enough dressing over the salad and toss to coat. Serve immediately.

Tropical Salad

6 Servings

Preparation time: 15 minutes

Ingredients

- ½ tsp minced garlic
- ½ tsp grated fresh ginger
- ¼ cup Olive oil
- ¼ tsp crushed Red pepper
- 3 tbsps Rice vinegar
- 3 tbsps Water
- 1 tbsp Soy sauce
- 2 cups Snow peas, sliced and blanched
- 3 Papayas, chopped
- 1 large carrot, shredded
- 1 Cucumber, peeled and sliced
- 3 cups shredded Romaine lettuce
- ½ cup chopped Roasted almonds
- Salt to taste

Directions

- Mix the garlic, ginger, olive oil, red pepper, vinegar, water, salt, and soy sauce in a bowl. Set aside.

- Add papaya, snow peas, cucumber slices, and carrot in a bowl.

- Sprinkle with the dressing and toss to coat.

- Place the lettuce on a plate and top with the salad.

- Now serve with the topping of almonds.

Mediterranean Pasta Salad

6 Servings

Preparation time: 15 minutes

Ingredients

- 8 oz Whole-Wheat pasta
- 1 (15.5-oz) can Chickpeas
- ½ cup Pitted Black olives
- ½ cup Minced Sun-dried tomatoes
- 1(6-oz) jar dill Pickles, sliced
- ½ cup Frozen peas, Thawed
- 1 tbsp capers
- 3 tsps dried chives
- ½ cup Olive oil
- 2 roasted red peppers, chopped
- ¼ cup White wine vinegar
- ½ tsp Dried basil
- 1 Garlic clove, minced
- Salt and Black pepper to taste

Directions

- Put some salt in water and add pasta in it and cook it for 8-10 minutes until all dente.

- Drain and put it into a bowl.

- Mix in chickpeas, olives, tomatoes, dill pickles, roasted peppers, peas, capers, and chives.

- Take another bowl, whisk oil, vinegar, basil, garlic, sugar, salt, and pepper.

- Pour over the pasta and toss to coat. Serve.

DINNER

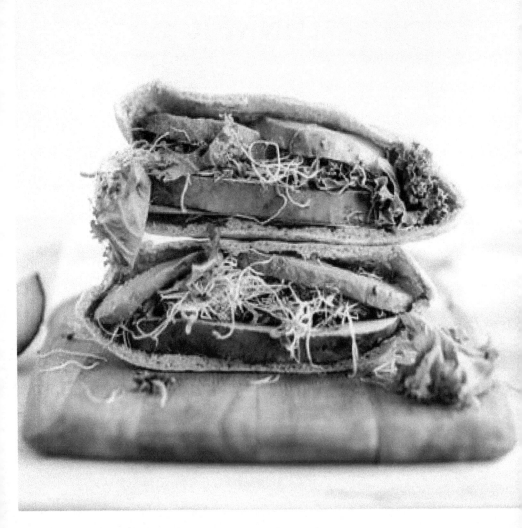

Veggie Paella with Lentils

6 Servings

Preparation Time: 50 minutes

Ingredients

- 2 tbsps Olive oil
- 3 cups Vegetable broth
- 1 ½ cups cooked Lentils, drained
- ¼ cup sliced pitted Black olives
- 2 tbsps minced fresh Parsley
- 1 Onion, chopped
- 1 Green bell pepper, chopped
- 2 Garlic cloves, minced
- 1 (14.5-oz) can diced Tomatoes
- 1 tbsp Capers
- ¼ tsp crushed red Pepper
- 1 ½ cups long-grain brown rice

Directions

- Heat oil in a pot over medium heat and sauté onion, bell pepper, and garlic for 5 minutes.
- Stir in tomatoes, capers, red pepper, and salt. Cook for 5 minutes. Pour in the rice and broth.
- Bring to a boil, then lower the heat.
- Simmer for 20 minutes.
- Turn the heat off and mix in lentils. Serve garnished with olives and parsley.

Paprika Cauliflower Tacos

8 Servings

Preparation Time: 40 minutes

Ingredients

- 1 head Cauliflower, cut into pieces
- Salt to taste
- 1 cup shredded Watercress
- 2 cups Cherry tomatoes, halved
- 2 Carrots, grated
- ½ cup Mango salsa
- ½ cup Guacamole
- 8 small Corn tortillas, warm
- 1 Lime, cut into wedges
- 2 tbsps Olive oil
- 2 tbsps Whole-wheat flour
- 2 tbsps nutritional Yeast
- 2 tsps Paprika
- 1 tsp Cayenne pepper

Directions

- Preheat oven to 350 F.

- Brush the cauliflower with oil in a bowl.

- In another bowl, mix the flour, yeast, paprika, cayenne pepper, and salt. Pour into the cauliflower bowl and toss to coat.

- Spread the cauliflower on a greased baking sheet. Bake for 20-30 minutes.

- In a bowl, combine the watercress, cherry tomatoes, carrots, mango salsa, and guacamole.

- Once the cauliflower is ready, divide it between the tortillas, add the mango mixture, roll up and serve with lime wedges on the side.

Simple Pesto Millet

6 Servings

Preparation Time: 50 minutes

Ingredients

- 1 cup Millet
- ½ cup Vegan basil pesto
- 2 ½ cups Vegetable broth

Directions

- Place the millet and broth in a pot.

- Bring to a boil, then lower the heat and simmer for 25 minutes.

- Let cool for 5 minutes and fluff the millet.

- Mix in the pesto and serve.

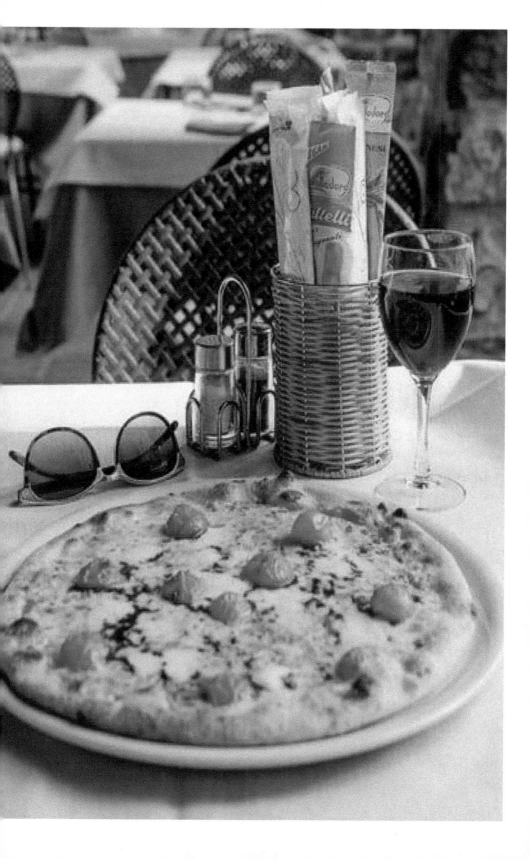

Peppered Pinto Beans

8 Servings

Preparation Time: 30 minutes

Ingredients

- 1 Serrano pepper, cut into strips
- 1 red Bell pepper, cut into strips
- 1 green Bell pepper, cut into strips
- 1 Onion, chopped
- 2 Carrots, chopped
- 2 Garlic cloves, minced
- 3 (15-oz) cans of pinto beans
- 18-ounce bottle Barbecue sauce
- ½ tsp Chipotle powder

Directions

- Place the serrano and bell peppers, onion, carrot, and garlic in a blender. Pulse until well mixed.

- Place the mixture in a pot with the beans, BBQ sauce, and chipotle powder. Cook for 15 minutes.

- Season with salt and pepper. Serve warm.

Black-Eyed Peas with Sun-Dried Tomatoes

6 Servings

Preparation Time: 35 minutes

Ingredients

- 1 cup Black-eyed peas, soaked overnight
- 1 tsp dried oregano
- ¾ tsp Garlic powder
- ½ tsp smoked paprika
- ¼ cup sun-dried Tomatoes, chopped
- 2 tbsps Olive oil
- 2 tsps ground chipotle pepper
- 1 ½ tsps ground Cumin
- 1 ½ tsps Onion powder

Directions

- Place the black-eyed peas in a pot and add 2 cups of water, olive oil, chipotle pepper, cumin, onion powder, oregano, garlic powder, salt, and paprika.

- Cook for 20 minutes over medium heat.

- Mix in sun-dried tomatoes, let sit for a few minutes and serve.

Vegetarian Quinoa Curry

6 Servings

Preparation Time: 35 minutes

Ingredients

- 4 tsps Olive oil
- 1 Onion, chopped
- 2 tbsps Curry powder
- 4 cups chopped spinach
- ½ cup non-dairy milk
- 2 tbsps Soy sauce
- Salt to taste
- 1 ½ cups quinoa
- 1 cup canned diced tomatoes

Directions

- Add oil into a pot and heat it over medium heat.

- Sauté the onion and ginger for 3 minutes until tender.

- Pour in curry powder, quinoa, and 3 cups of water. Bring to a boil, then lower the heat and simmer for 15-20 minutes.

- Mix in tomatoes, spinach, milk, soy sauce, and salt.

- Simmer for an additional 3 minutes.

Alfredo Rice with Green Beans

4 Servings

Preparation Time: 25 minutes

Ingredients

- 1 cup Alfredo arugula vegan pesto
- 2 cups brown rice
- 1 cup frozen green beans, thawed

Directions

- Cook the rice in salted water in a pot over medium heat for 20 minutes.

- Drain and let it cool completely.

- Place the Alfredo sauce and beans in a skillet.

- Cook over low heat for 3-5 minutes.

- Mix in the rice to coat. Serve immediately.

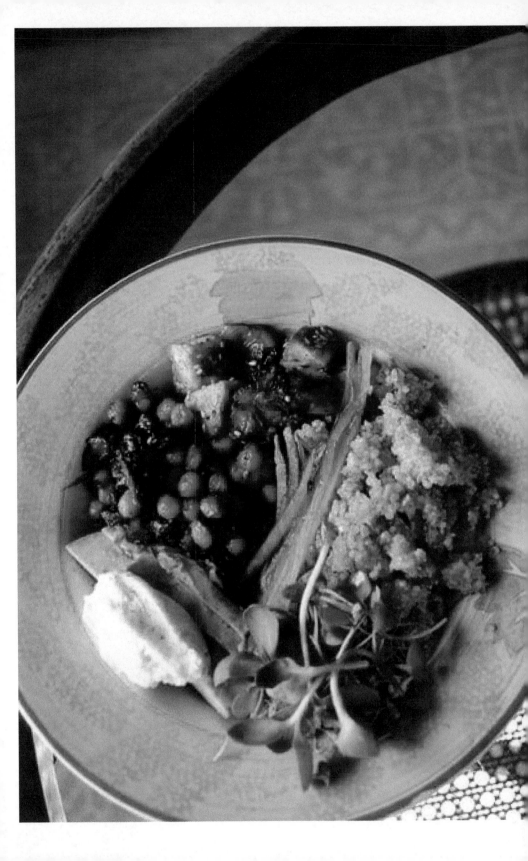

Korean-Style Millet

6 Servings

Preparation Time: 30 minutes

Ingredients

- 1 cup dried Millet, drained
- Salt and Black pepper to taste
- 1 tsp Gochugaru flakes

Directions

- Place the millet and gochugaru flakes in a pot.

- Cover with enough water and bring to a boil.

- Lower the heat and simmer for 20 minutes. Drain and let cool.

- Transfer to a serving bowl and season with salt and pepper. Serve.

DESSERTS

Mixed Berry Yogurt Ice Pops

6 Servings

Preparation Time: 5 minutes

Ingredients

- 2/3 cup avocado, halved and pitted
- 2/3 cup frozen berries, thawed
- 1 cup dairy-free yogurt
- ½ cup coconut cream
- 1 tsp vanilla extract

Directions

- Pour the avocado pulp, berries, dairy-free yogurt, coconut cream, and vanilla extract.

- Process until smooth. Pour into ice pop sleeves and freeze for 8 or more hours.

- Enjoy the ice pops when ready.

Holiday Pecan Tart

4 Servings

Preparation Time: 50 minutes

Ingredients

- 4 tbsps flaxseed powder
- 1/3 cup whole-wheat flour
- ½ tsp salt
- ¼ cup cold plant butter, crumbled
- 3 tbsps pure malt syrup

For the filling:
- 3 tbsps flaxseed powder + 9 tbsps water
- 2 cups toasted pecans, chopped
- 1 cup light corn syrup
- ½ cup pure date sugar
- 1 tbsp pure pomegranate molasses
- 4 tbsps plant butter, melted
- ½ tsp salt
- 2 tsps vanilla extract

Directions

- Preheat oven to 350 F. In a bowl, mix the flaxseed powder with 12 tbsps water and allow thickening for 5 minutes. Do this for the filling's vegan "flax egg" too in a separate bowl.

- In a bowl, combine flour and salt. Add in plant butter and whisk until crumbly. Pour in the crust's vegan "flax egg" and maple syrup and mix until smooth dough forms.

- Flatten the dough on a flat surface, cover with plastic wrap, and refrigerate for 1 hour. Dust a working surface with flour, remove the dough onto the surface, and using a rolling pin, flatten the dough into a 1-inch diameter circle.

- Lay the dough on a greased pie pan and press to fit the shape of the pan. Trim the edges of the pan.

- Lay a parchment paper on the dough, pour on some baking beans and bake for 20 minutes. Remove, pour out baking beans, and allow cooling.

- In a bowl, mix the filling's vegan "flax egg," pecans, corn syrup, date sugar, pomegranate molasses, plant butter, salt, and vanilla.

- Pour and spread the mixture on the piecrust. Bake for 20 minutes or until the filling sets.

- Remove from the oven, decorate with more pecans, slice, and cool. Slice and serve.

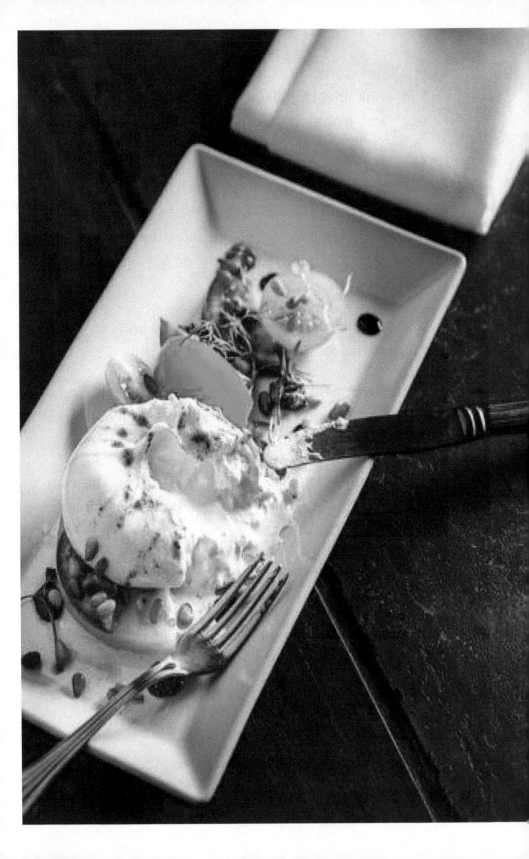

Coconut Chocolate Barks

4 Servings

Preparation Time: 35 minutes

Ingredients

- 1/3 cup coconut oil, melted
- ¼ cup almond butter, melted
- 2 tbsps unsweetened coconut flakes.
- 1 tsp pure maple syrup
- A pinch of ground rock salt
- ¼ cup unsweetened cocoa nibs

Directions

- Line a baking tray with baking paper and set aside. In a medium bowl, mix the coconut oil, almond butter, coconut flakes, maple syrup, and fold in the rock salt and cocoa nibs.

- Pour and spread the mixture on the baking sheet, chill in the refrigerator for 20 minutes or until firm.

- Remove the dessert, break into shards, and enjoy. Preserve extras in the refrigerator.

Nutty Date Cake

4 Servings

Preparation Time: 1 hour 30 minutes

Ingredients

- ½ cup cold plant butter, cut into pieces
- 1 tbsp flaxseed powder
- ½ cup whole-wheat flour
- ¼ cup chopped pecans and walnuts
- 1 tsp baking powder
- 1 tsp baking soda
- 1 tsp cinnamon powder
- 1 tsp salt
- 1/3 cup pitted dates, chopped
- ½ cup pure date sugar
- 1 tsp vanilla extract
- ¼ cup pure date syrup for drizzling.

Directions

- Preheat oven to 350 F and lightly grease a baking dish with some plant butter.

- In a small bowl, mix the flaxseed powder with 3 tbsps water and allow thickening for 5 minutes to make the vegan "flax egg."

- In a food processor, add the flour, nuts, baking powder, baking soda, cinnamon powder, and salt.

- Blend until well combined. Add 1/3 cup of water, dates, date sugar, and vanilla. Process until smooth with tiny pieces of dates evident.

- Pour the batter into the baking dish and bake in the oven for 1 hour and 10 minutes or until a toothpick inserted comes out clean.

- Remove the dish from the oven, invert the cake onto a serving platter to cool, drizzle with the date syrup, slice, and serve.

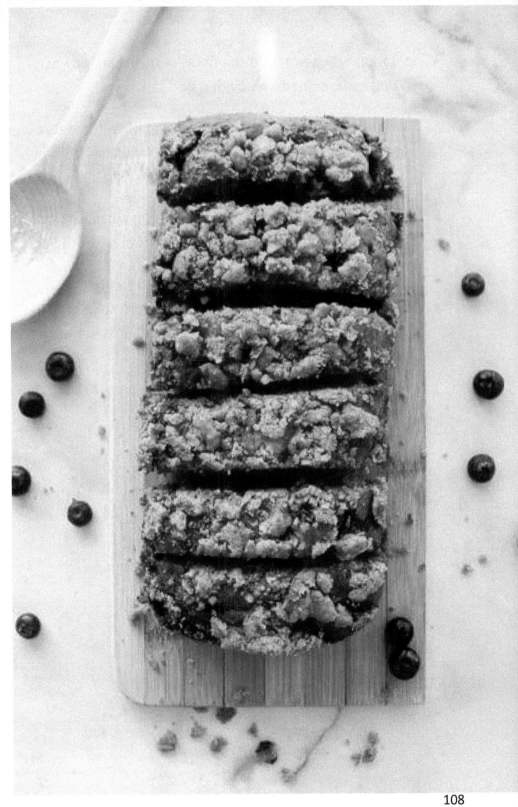

Berry Cupcakes with Cashew Cheese Icing

4 Servings

Preparation Time: 35 minutes

Ingredients

- 2 cups whole-wheat flour
- ¼ cup cornstarch
- 2 ½ tsps baking powder
- 1 ½ cups pure date sugar
- ½ tsp salt
- ¾ cup plant butter, softened
- 3 tsps vanilla extract
- 1 cup strawberries, pureed
- 1 cup oat milk, room temperature
- ¾ cup cashew cream
- 2 tbsps coconut oil, melted
- 3 tbsps pure maple syrup
- 1 tsp vanilla extract
- 1 tsp freshly squeezed lemon juice

Directions

- Preheat the oven to 350 F and line a 12-holed muffin tray with cupcake liners. Set aside.

- In a bowl, mix flour, cornstarch, baking powder, date sugar, and salt. Whisk in plant butter, vanilla extract, strawberries, and oat milk until well combined.

- Divide the mixture into the muffin cups two-thirds way up and bake for 20-25 minutes. Allow cooling while you make the frosting.

- In a blender, add cashew cream, coconut oil, maple syrup, vanilla, and lemon juice.

- Process until smooth. Pour the frosting into a medium bowl and chill for 30 minutes.

- Transfer the mixture into a piping bag and swirl mounds of the frosting onto the cupcakes.

- Serve immediately.

Coconut & Chocolate Cake

4 Servings

Preparation Time: 40 minutes

Ingredients

- 2/3 cup toasted almond flour
- ¼ cup unsalted plant butter, melted
- 2 cups chocolate bars, cubed
- 2 ½ cups coconut cream
- Fresh berries for topping

Directions

- Lightly grease a 9-inch springform pan with some plant butter and set it aside.

- Mix the almond flour and plant butter in a medium bowl and pour the mixture into the springform pan. Use the spoon to spread and press the mixture into the bottom of the pan. Place in the refrigerator to firm for 30 minutes.

- Meanwhile, pour the chocolate in a safe microwave bowl and melt for 1 minute stirring every 30 seconds. Remove from the microwave and mix in the coconut cream and maple syrup.

- Remove the cake pan from the oven, pour the chocolate mixture on top, and shake the pan and even the layer. Chill further for 4 to 6 hours. Take out the pan from the fridge, release the cake and garnish with the raspberries or strawberries. Slice and serve.

Lightning Source UK Ltd.
Milton Keynes UK
UKHW020707130521
383649UK00005B/42

9 781802 853896